Alzheimer's

Observations & Disclosures & Resolutions

by

Harlan Carl Scheffler

GR

George Ronald
Oxford

George Ronald, *Publisher*
Oxford
www.grbooks.com

*A catalogue record for this book is available
from the British Library*

ISBN 978–0–85398–553–2

Contents

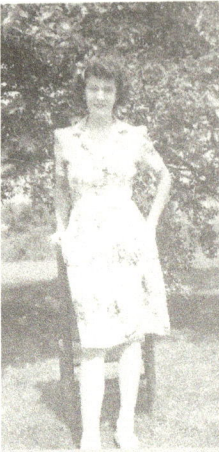

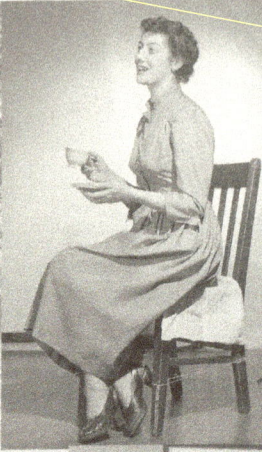

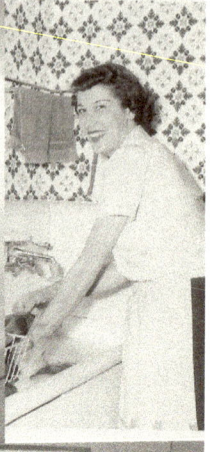

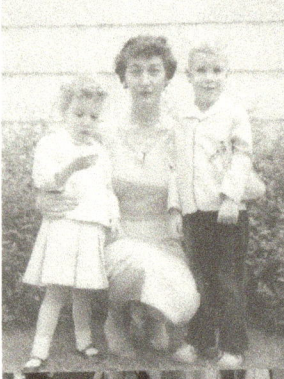

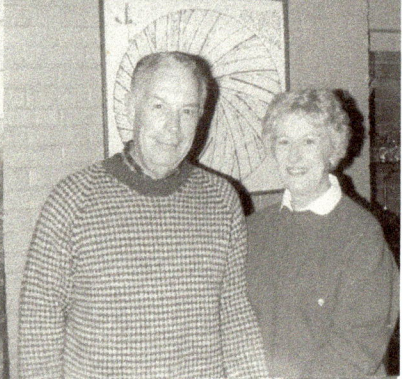

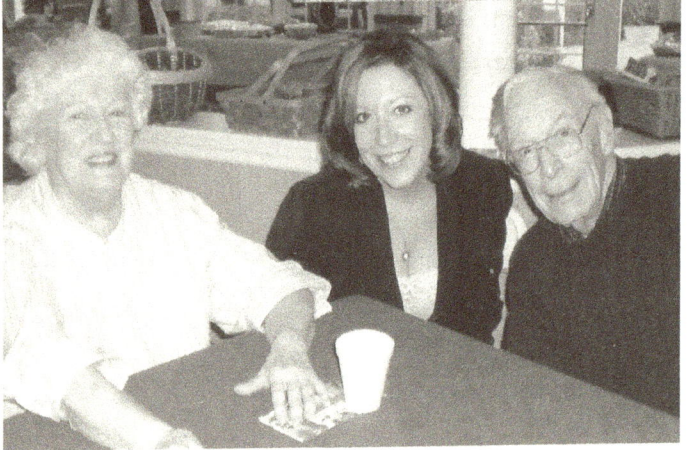

Part One

My Alzheimer's

My birthday was May 17, 1926. For some reason Harlan likes to pretend he is older than he is by marking his arrival time nine months before his birthday; he's like that – makes things more complicated than they are. Calvin Coolidge was then president and a first class postage stamp cost two cents. I was born in Indianapolis, Indiana. My sister, Mary Ellen, preceded me by three years. I was a tomboy, better at baseball than with paper dolls. My family was Quaker, so early on I found happiness going to Meeting and growing up with other Friends who were friends. My dad called me Pud, though I'm not sure why. Maybe I was his li'l puddin'. I was a good student except for spelling: one time when I was at Quaker Camp I wrote home that I 'slud' into first base.

When I was nine I got rheumatic fever and had to stay in bed for a year. Then I went to cripple school. Unfortunately, I casually mentioned to my family that I knew a boy at school whose name was Salvatore Screwy. Apparently some people don't have enough to do. Harlan and the kids couldn't let it rest and fantasized that if had I married Salvatore we could have named our daughter Lucy. Ha, ha. Anyway, I got better.

In Indianapolis my father worked at many jobs. The late twenties were dark times. No steady work. We moved nine times, sometimes staying with relatives. For years my mother's mother, Grandma Ball, rented out rooms and served meals to laborers, and late in her life she daily rode a bus to Fort Benjamin Harrison to do laundry and work in the kitchen. Her husband had left her years earlier. He was a ladies' man and a drinker. My dad's dad died when he was 35, and Leanora, my other grandmother, was not much good after that. Her older son, Glenn, looked after her. He owned a big dry cleaning and laundry business. Dad worked for him until he and mom packed up and moved to Chicago. Somewhere in there dad got into the extract business – flavorings for soft drinks. Mom worked at L.S. Ayers department store – she was good in retail, curtains, etc.

The move was awful. I was 19. I was lost in Chicago. I left all my friends in Indianapolis. I tried junior college: not good. Mom thought I would be a good model, so I went to Patricia Stevens Agency and was then hired by one of Chicago's large commercial art studios. Harlan's sister was a fashion illustrator there and she arranged for the two of us to meet at a beach party in Wilmette on the shore of Lake Michigan. I wore red shorts, a red polka dot white blouse and a red floppy hat. I had a sunburned nose and Harlan said later that I was cute as a button. We were married in 1951.

Harlan used to say that when he first met my mom and dad he 'knew he was marrying into money'. In our tiny house on Meade Avenue, mom, wearing her pink robe and matching mule slippers, was lying on the couch in our living room. I don't remember such a tale. He exaggerates. Maybe she had a cold. Anyway, he was right: he did not marry for money – or apparently he didn't, because we are still married. Like his dad and my own dad, Harlan worked hard all his life. Together, over 57 years, we bought three homes, raised two fine children, and saved enough money to live three years in this assisted care facility.

I guess it's just the luck of the Irish–Scottish–English–French that I have Alzheimer's. It seems to attack indiscriminately. Its signs appear so subtly that we are unaware that what is happening is happening. But, then, life is a fragile business no matter what our circumstances.

Although Harlan is writing my story, this *is* my story. I probably should have started with our first meeting with George and Marilyn. This was years ago when Harlan and I were newly married. The four of us would meet at state parks in Indiana and Illinois and Michigan, and we would tramp the trails and have fun after supper playing Kings in the Corner or dominos. We would recall the good times and laugh at the same stories – how we met over drinks at the bar. Ha, ha. Actually we were introduced at a religious gathering in a second floor rented meeting room above a tavern, the jukebox downstairs thumping loudly: ♪'Don't fence me in. Let me ride through the wide open country that I love, don't fence me in.'♪

One evening, about six or seven years ago, we were playing dominos and I seemed to be having trouble. I would match the six dots alongside the four. We all laughed when we saw my mistake.

'We better watch Barb; she's a sly one.'

I didn't have a clue that there was something different going on – if there was. However, over the following weeks and months I gradually lost interest in my jigsaw puzzles and those word-find puzzle books. Reading became tedious. I would read the same words over and over and the story would never get anyplace. United States history, the Civil War – these were my favorite subjects. On those getaway weekends with George and Marilyn, Harlan and I would search the small town byways for quaint bookshops and we would look on the dusty shelves for forgotten editions about Lincoln and Mary Todd and Gettysburg. I had quite a collection. And we were always on the lookout for antique perfume bottles.

'Hey, Barb, over here; here's a pretty one that's different.'

I had over a hundred. They were so beautiful – some were crystal with subtle blue and purple tints.

Progressively over the years I was having trouble with ordinary, familiar activities. A few summers ago I lost interest in planting and tending the garden. Traditionally, our garden up by the road was so beautiful passersby would honk and wave as they drove past, and there were two occasions when, on seeing me working, they turned into our driveway and thanked me for the flowers. They were total strangers. All that gradually passed away. Ironing our clothes, turning on the washing machine or microwave, operating the dishwasher and adjusting the thermostat became impossible. I put socks in the sugar bowl. I could not speak coherently. People who were not familiar with my illness would ask me, 'What did you say?' but I would not be able even to recall what sparked my motivation to speak. It was like living in a nether world, neither here nor there. It is not like a dream where you are totally involved with the sequence of events and when the events take a nasty turn you say, 'Enough of that, I think I'll wake up.' Or like a daydream where you sit quietly and then drift off into another world, and then you come back. With Alzheimer's you can't come back.

Harlan used to tell (what he thought was) a funny story. Some few years ago he underwent surgery. Dr Hrisomolos repaired a hole in the retinal tissue of his right eye. Under anesthetic Harlan was drifting in and out of consciousness and at times he could vaguely hear the nurses and attendants idly talking. One said that he saw on television that wild creatures, after giving birth to their young, tidy up the delivery room by eating the placenta. Another attendant thought it should be shared that very primitive human societies most likely did the same thing. Everyone said, 'Ugh!' Harlan interjected, with a wispy, detached voice, 'Depends on how you fix it.' Funny? Well, perhaps maybe, but even though he was fuzzy, he was still connected to this world.

Now, I'm folding and unfolding my napkin, frantically, obsessively smoothing and brushing my place mat, constantly touching and moving silverware and water glasses, pouring coffee into my oatmeal and orange juice on the floor. I wonder where my coffee is as I drink it. This is my breakfast, lunch and dinner – unless I have my Trazodone. I have been on Aricept and Namenda for three years and these medications have shown, only perhaps, that they slow down the debilitating repercussions of my Alzheimer's. They say Trazodone helps stem the anxiety that comes over me during the course of the day and night. At these times I can hardly stay still, I must move about – my energy seems to spin off in all directions. After these occurrences I do not remember them.

The literature says that Alzheimer's is most often diagnosed early on with signs of short-term memory loss. Four years ago my first appointment with a neurologist clearly disclosed that I had lost much of my short- and long-term recall. I could not tell the time of day by looking at a clock, nor could I draw a circle and place clock numbers in it. Or write my name. My town and my state, the season of the year – all lost. But sometimes earlier childhood impressions did and do flash back. I now ask Harlan, 'Could we phone mom and dad tonight?' And this will trigger, 'Have you heard from Mary Ellen?' though my sister died nine years ago. The old memories and current events get mixed up. Casually looking out the dining room window at the fire station across the road, I pat my napkin and venture to say, 'The horses are all folded.' Am I recalling a story my father used to tell?

> I heard a terrible ruckus, bells clanging and people shouting as a horse-drawn fire engine raced past me. The horses were very close – frenzied, out of control – and I could see their wild bloodshot eyes and flared nostrils. As they sped by, puffing, one lost his footing, slipped and fell right in front of me. I could see the marks of his flesh on the bricks afterwards.

Seeing the fire station and patting my napkin. Were the horses all safe and put away for the night?

At the time of this writing Harlan and I have been here in this assisted care residence for almost three years. We left our log cabin in the woods hurriedly because an 'apartment' was available here, and, as our kids, Todd and Nancy, and their families are living nearby, they could help with the intricacies of such a move. And it was a fitting move, even though we left friends and surroundings, timely because Harlan and I were really not able to take care of my needs as we did, even weeks earlier, back there in Nashville.

Now I am spending my days in the Reminiscence. Here, the very caring care managers devote their time to keeping me safe. I feel more secure; everything is scaled down so that I am not overwhelmed with high ceilings and open spaces. I am surrounded by old pictures and things that I might remember as a child growing up. Over here is the Philco radio my mom and dad had in their living room. There's mom's mirror. Mom made all these napkins. I love to fold them. See?

Part Two

Our Story Unfolds

When Barbara and I were living in Nashville, Indiana, sort of tucked away in a cabin in the woods, we were at home with nature. The squirrels and chipmunks and deer were our neighbors. We counted some 30 different bird species and we had bluebird and wren houses all through the near woods. Hummingbirds returned each spring on April 14 or 15 and then, on their designated day in the fall, they bade us farewell with like accord. Our log house was a storybook home. Guests would step inside and pause to breathe in some vague recollection they had of the past. Our furnishings were old family pieces and antiques. Kerosene lamps adorned the walls. I recall some years ago I thought it would be interesting to learn how to spin yarn. The historical society gave me an old wheel and I can still see our images – Barbara knitting by the fireplace, and me, over there in the corner carding some wool and pedaling the treadle, a perfect addition – except when I occasionally looked up from my snags to watch the news of the day on TV.

We thought that the move from Chicago to Brown County in southern Indiana would be our last move – a retreat from long years of paying attention to business. Both our children and their families were living in Cincinnati and I suppose we could have moved closer to them but, as we all say, 'They have their own lives to live', and besides, Barbara and I were still in somewhat prime condition. We lived in that idyllic setting for 20 years.

Some of my commercial art clients saw no trouble in continuing to feed jobs my way so we added a studio to one of the back bedrooms. Barbara found work right away. She was good, very good, at retail sales – like her mother. The owners of small shops sought her service. The Print Shop, The Toy Chest, The Book Loft, The Family Tree all wanted her. Even earlier, back home in Chicago, Creative Gift and Slocum's Children's Shop customers would enter the store and ask for Barbara to help them choose the right wedding gift or party dress.

Moving from DuPage County to Brown County, leaving

the big city – and all that is wrapped up in it – to live in so rural a setting was perhaps preset early in both our lives, years before we met. Barbara grew up in Indianapolis but did not find tranquility, perhaps not even true happiness, until her family moved to Hunter Road out in the country. Her father befriended the hardpan clay soil until, after a few seasons of caring, he could harvest potatoes with his bare hands. Barbara and her mother canned hundreds of jars of green beans and corn and tomatoes season after season. To earn a little extra money during the depression years, the family raised chickens and sold them, dressed and ready for roasting, to neighbors and friends from church. Barbara was three years younger than her sister Mary Ellen so she had the job of cleaning the chicken coop, scalding the chickens and plucking the feathers – albeit nasty work, but this was country living, and this was where she was happiest.

As she tells her story, it is clear that her family's move to Chicago was not a free choice; rather it was the consequence of her father's dedication to work. He was a chemist, learned his trade on the job and eventually formulated his own recipes for soft drink flavors. His raspberry punch was special. Barbara occasionally would tell us the story of her family's arrival at the Greyhound bus depot, suitcases in hand, and how they then rode the 'red-rattler' streetcar to a house that they had never seen – purchased by the company he was to work for. Meade Avenue was a Timbuktu jump from Hunter Road.

I too loved the out-of-doors. Early on, when I was just a youngster, riding my bicycle to the forest preserve to poke around in the ponds and streams was a happy time. Looking for a vacation spot in the woods, my folks found 'Rismon's' in a magazine advertisement and year after year we went back to the Lodge on Ballard Lake in northern Wisconsin to tramp the old logging trails. At the close of each day, tucked into beds on lumpy mattresses, we listened for the haunting call of the loon. And this ritual continued with Barbara and me and our kids until they married. Barbie and I have had a wonderful life together. Over all those 57 years, every Friday night was our date night.

Back in those earlier years, neither of us knew anything about Alzheimer's. But then it was not a household word. Dementia was the one that lurked in the shadows. Both our parents were perhaps a shade away from hale and hearty but they were active and full of life. Barbara's folks lived long lives. Her father was 96 and her mother 85. In my own family, I cannot remember my mother ever going to a doctor. I do recall, when I was very young, traipsing off to the hospital to visit a relative, Aunt Mazie, who was recovering from an operation – and I thought she was very old – probably she was somewhere around fifty and a half. I think the visit made a lasting impression on me because she unceremoniously showed us what I think was her goiter floating in a bottle next to her bed.

I didn't know any of my grandparents but Barbara knew all of hers, so she was better acquainted with the process of people getting old. They, all four, completed their tour of duty with, apparently, no signs of Alzheimer's or other dementias. However, whatever the subtle signs of 'senility' might have been evident then would probably be more objectively diagnosed today.

I have tried to trace back and pick out some early signs of Barbara's illness. In high school Barbara was president of the Penguin Club and was so outgoing and straightforward and good-hearted to be named May Queen – an extraordinary happening in that she had just transferred from another school district. Some of the other girls' mothers were not too happy about this very unfortunate turn of events. I learned that through her earlier years, even before our marriage, she occasionally lost her sense of taste and smell. I do not know if this means anything. Occasionally she suffered severe migraine headaches but she had no chronic health problems. When we were first married she was very active in the good-works agenda of the Tri-Kappa sorority, attending meetings, serving on committees and enthusiastically entering into the various activities with the 'girls'. However, she did not go out alone on these occasions. I drove her to the meeting place and then, by myself, had supper with a book. Our two children were born a year apart, so during their growing up years Barbara became a stay-at-home mom. She was an ideal new mother. All in all, she was (and is) a most open and loveable individual. She attracted everyone; her genuine kindness and goodness touched all who knew her. She was captain of the local chapter of the National Cerebral Palsy Association – took our two little kids with her on her door-to-door campaign.

It was perhaps after the children set out for college that her self assurance seemed to fade, but then she was never ever overbearing. She then appeared to be more comfortable relying on my judgment and initiative, and I gradually learned that I had a more responsible role to play in our marriage. I would take the first step and Barbie would be content to follow. This was not the case when it came time to bake her famous birthday cake or chocolate brownies with 'gooey' sauce. And, throughout our marriage, up to about three years ago, she would sort through the recipe cards and bake hundreds of intricate Christmas cookies, made with painstaking love – and butter – to give as gifts to neighbors and friends. However, it was understood that I would take the present to the door and ring the bell. Barbie would wave her greeting from the car. Over later months and years I was doing more of the shopping for groceries and donning the apron to prepare our meals. However, it did provoke a ruffle when I washed the dishes in the kitchen sink, believing the dishwasher used too much hot water. Barbara liked the silver and glassware to glisten and sparkle.

I think it was about four years ago that Barbara was working at the bookstore and she was having trouble making change for the customers. They would reach over the counter to help her count out the right coins for their overpayment. Oftentimes we would bring home the day's sales receipts and would try to figure out what was what and then fill in the daily record – adding a dollar or two to make it all tally. Finally the store owner, a dear friend, confided that Barbara was getting too confused to carry on. Although she missed this activity – the working and the meeting with people, which she always liked – she acquiesced, perhaps with a hint of understanding, though I am not sure. She had fun at her retirement party and never mentioned or indicated an awareness of the decline of her capacities; but, then, she always looked for the positive side of things and shied away from negative thinking.

Some few weeks later I accompanied Barbara to her doctor's office and we both waited in the examining room. Being there with her, I could help answer some of the questions that might be asked. I mentioned to the doctor that Barbie had been experiencing dizziness and occasionally fainting spells and she would have to sit or lie down for a few minutes until they passed; that one time I heard and felt a serious thump in the kitchen and, rushing in, I found Barbara on the floor trembling and shaking, though she seemed to be unconscious. I held her for a few minutes until she recovered her presence of mind. Her doctor prescribed Namenda and Aricept but the dizziness and fainting spells became more frequent as the weeks ran on. Her doctor referred her to a neurologist and after four or five appointments, where the same preliminary questions were asked – 'Do you know what day this is?' 'Can you tell me the season of the year?' 'Do you know the name of your town?' – she underwent MRI and CAT scan procedures, and her illness was confirmed as Alzheimer's disease. At this point, Barbara did not understand what this meant. We had never ever talked about Alzheimer's.

At any rate, as Barbara became more detached from her normal life, her friends and surroundings, we decided to make the move to Cincinnati, Ohio, where our children and their families still lived. Throughout this whole drama she shared only once her awareness of what was happening. Entering our new home, surveying the 'grandeur' of this assisted living facility, she voiced clear and certain – 'I'm so sorry . . . for all of this' – and her hand futilely swept across the room. I suddenly found I was crying. I tear a bit as I write these words.

Moving into an assisted living facility is traumatic. There is no way to describe what happens to the individual when she or he is given cause to leave everything behind – to get rid of everything. Certainly in our case, Barbara could not know fully why we were moving. I tried to prepare her for the dreaded moment when we would close the door to our cabin, get into our son's car and drive away. The last year of our residence in Nashville, the weeks and months that confirmed the necessity of such a move, revolved entirely around Barbara's needs. Increasingly I found that I could not do what needed to be done to compensate for the debilitating effects that Alzheimer's was imposing on her. Some of our friends questioned why I was going with Barbara, that '. . . there's a nice community nursing home right here in Nashville. You could visit Barbie as often as you would like and still stay here'. Somehow I never considered this as an option. I would have to go with her, and the assisted living center could supply accommodation for both of us.

Moving into a two-room apartment in such a facility is difficult. Trying to care for Barbara in this new environment – explaining what it is that we are doing – is difficult. And then moving Barbie to Reminiscence, the adjacent Alzheimer's unit, after being together for just six months, was difficult – for both of us. I am reminded of M. Scott Peck's worthy book *The Road Less Traveled*. Dr Peck's opening theme is most relevant. Life is difficult; once you know this, it becomes less difficult. Now, when I am not with Barbara, she often asks about me: 'Have you seen Harlan?' She is aware that I am not with her and therefore I must be someplace else. The care managers tell me that she keeps busy walking, strolling around the premises, pausing to gaze at the garden, moving small objects from here to there and sometimes just sitting alone or with friends. We have supper together most every evening. When I enter the dining room, I drag in her old world with me. She looks up and smiles and, with special effort, voices, 'Hi honey. Is that you? Have you heard from mom and dad? And Mary Ellen, did she call? Where's the car? Where have you been? Are we going to sleep together tonight?'

When I first see her, before she sees me, she is sitting quietly, holding a piece of knitted material or a page from a magazine. When I am not with her she seems to be content. It is when I am with her that she becomes confused and tries to tie things together. When the residents in Reminiscence have a party or there is a special program, Barbara enters in with sheer joy. Sherrill told me she was singing and dancing the hokey pokey – completely unaware of herself. She was laughing and making funny faces to the music – exaggerated smiles and scowls – just having fun. Increasingly, her world is becoming more complete as she leaves mine. If I had been there, I would have put a damper on the whole affair, I'm quite sure. When we were youngsters, long before we met, Barb was the bobby-sock-saddle-shoed teenager out there with the crowd, jitter-bugging her heart out. I would have been the quiet chap over there in the corner sipping my Coke, waiting for the 'one step' to start. So I am not sure what role I am playing now because she seems to be better off when I am not there – even though she is asking about me. It would seem that some of the other residents are hardly aware of the comings and goings of their relatives and friends. Barb has not reached this stage yet. It is a most difficult time. However, there is one consideration, a question that we cannot avoid. When a dear one is so ravaged with Alzheimer's that he or she is not able to express normal feelings and reactions, can we assume that these feelings and a certain private condition of awareness are not still there, held secret? It is an important consideration. What if the ones closest to you decide to go away – and stay away – and you 'somehow' know it?

This morning's post brought me a note from Gineen, one of the care managers in Reminiscence. She is a wonderful young woman from Ghana. She wrote, in her own manner of speech, 'Barbara is a real sweet person. She real concerned about the resident. She like to make sure they get there meal. She like to look at Books. She like to join in activity by doing exercise and she like singing. She a real sweet person.'

Now, as I write, Barbara is most likely walking the halls or perhaps sitting quietly alone. In just a little while, I will visit with her and we will have supper together. She will be happy to see me and she will ask about our car and about her sister. She will need help with her food. It will appear that she does not quite know what to do with it. Sometimes when I prepare a serving, Barbie will pick up the spoon – but, oftentimes, not. At 86, I feel my own dexterity is fading; I am not as quick as I used to be. It's amazing how fast a noodle or meatball or strawberry shortcake can find its way into one's coffee – anyone's coffee.

In the books and articles that explore the ramifications of Alzheimer's, there is considerable mention of the toll that is inflicted on the family. I believe the general consensus is that the family must take care that they are not so burdened with feelings of helplessness and guilt that they are not able to bring happiness to their loved one. I have found that my state of mind definitely connects with Barbara's. She will sense that I am distracted or she will be cheered with my good humor. She is troubled enough without having to share my concerns. As she eats her supper, I rub and scratch her back and hum 'yummy' sounds. Immediately she is in a state of rapture. Sighing and smiling, she closes her eyes. The more frequently I am with her, the less is her need to adjust to my sudden departure and reappearance, even though she does not remember how long ago it was that I was with her. As we sit together, the music playing softly in the background, Barbara will whisper the tune – right on key – and be happy. Barbara is my teacher. I suddenly find that I am happy too.

Last evening we were sitting at the supper table with her friends and I reminisced about our dating days, how we went to the symphony concerts and ballet, even saw Rudolf Nureyev and Margot Fonteyn in Chicago; that one time Barbara said, 'Harlan, you're spending an awful lot of money on me!' and I thought, 'Hmm, she's right' and, to put a stop to it, I married her. Lillian laughed and Barbie smiled and threatened me with her rolled-up napkin. Then, as her gaze drifted, she voiced, 'I was a peach growing on the tree until I was plucked.' When I pass Patrick, busily preparing the food in the kitchen, he laughs and greets me with his charming accent, 'Ah, Harlan, you are going to have a dining experience.' I laugh too. He is so right.

Part Three

The Nature of Things

Brain, Mind, Soul and Spirit

Since Barbara's illness was diagnosed, I have read numerous articles and books about Alzheimer's. I have attended lectures and seminars and support groups, studied Internet postings, trying to bring the reality of what is happening to the level of my understanding. The information that is available is voluminous. I have tried to glean knowledge of the workings of the human brain so that, as a layman, I am not a mere onlooker but in some degree a participant in this whole scenario. There are innumerable Internet websites devoted to sharing data about dementia and Alzheimer's, as well as thousands of books and articles describing both scientific findings and psychological points of view. We are generally persuaded to place our trust in hard-fact scientific research because this approach to knowledge has proven to be practical and successful over the years. So many debilitating illnesses and disabilities have been defined, treated and in many cases cured through the instrumentation of science.

However, focusing on the brain and its function, when viewed from a purely scientific perspective, employing clinical testing and experiment, then arriving at explainable propositions, cannot but harbor a bit of uncertainty. The structure of the brain, its various lobe configurations and nerve centers and then the miraculous behavior of this simple physical matter – atoms of elements, molecules of atoms, and cells of molecules that make up the brain – might easily rob us of some of our certainty. How is it that this physical substance *behaves?* In my search for answers, this is the most important of all my questions: What causes matter to toe the line? The relationship of the physical brain to its astounding function is less than straightforward.

Throughout my adult life I have endeavored to construct a foundation for understanding. I have long felt, perhaps intuitively, that certainty does not exclusively rest on rational proofs. When I read about the function of the brain and the toll Alzheimer's takes when it creeps into a life, I immediately weigh the findings and the arrived-at conclusions against my personal assessment of 'truth' and I ask myself, 'Does this fit? Does this make sense?'

The research that is being done on Alzheimer's is widespread. There is an urgency to find a cause of this debilitating disease and then a cure or treatment because the world's population is growing fast. Many of us old folks are living longer and there are countless young people who are now unwittingly in harm's way. I am impatient. Because of the urgent need for answers to Alzheimer's perplexing questions, I am compelled to look outside the normal scientific fields of inquiry for explanations and clarifications, particularly because there is a real possibility that the current search agenda may not insure that conclusive answers are in the offing. The present inquiry establishes a boundary line that outlaws a more comprehensive search and this may be the very obstacle that suppresses the achievement of the coveted goal. As untutored as I may be in the disciplines of modern research and technology, I am advantaged in being free to investigate reasonable propositions that heretofore have not been acknowledged but today might prove to be sound. Therefore I submit this essay for your consideration, for I suspect it may not, quite yet, find a hearing ear in today's scientific community.

This basis for confidence may at first appear to be a naive trust and I have no defense to plead. It is just that, when examining causes and effects in the light of rational thought, certain conclusions are unavoidable. It would appear that the whole of life is made up of consequences – one thing causing another thing to happen. This networking could easily be designated a universal or natural law. If this law of causes and effects has universal application, then it must be deemed relevant not only in the material world but in the spiritual world as well. Practical science's longstanding dilemma is that it cannot recognize the totality of life – its material *and* its non-material aspects – and then their correspondence. This equation is a constant. For example: In the material world we plant seeds and water them and they grow into viable plants – so that we might have food to eat and air to breathe. A storm rages, a tree falls to the ground – so that life can be made new. These causes and effects are inseparable. And in (what we call) the spiritual world, we plant intangible seeds: a friend is heartbroken and we respond with earnest compassion – so that human love can find expression and grow. You smile and give a gift, say, a coin of some value, to a total stranger – without looking back – and the two of you will never be the same. It is irrefutable: both the physical and spiritual aspects of our humanity are self-evident and proven.

When I was working in a commercial art studio in Chicago I had a friend who was a lettering artist. Vic and his wife Gwen and their daughter Emily were campers – they too loved the woods and state parks. One Friday night of a holiday weekend Vic had to work late and this upset the family's plan. They had hoped to leave early and arrive at the campsite before the evening hours. When he finally got home, Gwen and Emily were all packed and ready, so off they went to the park. They arrived at the gate to find the guard in a worrisome mood. He had had a day of it. Vic explained that they had planned to get there earlier but he had had to work, etc.

Exasperated, perspiring, visibly distraught, the attendant angrily replied, 'What do you want me to do about that? All the camping spots are taken, you're out of luck, there's no room for you!'

Emily, who has Down's syndrome, leaned forward from the back seat and poked her head out of Vic's window. Interrupting the guard's tantrum, she said, 'What's your name?'

He stopped short.

'Err, ah, George. What's yours?'

'I'm Emily.'

The guard lifted his gaze towards the campground and said, 'Well, let's see now. Where can we put you folks?'

Little Emily disarmed the guard. The eight year old could have had no idea that she would be my teacher, that she would enhance my life – and now, possibly, yours – but not in any tangible way. Rather, in a way far more meaningful and profound.

It would be foolish to pretend that I have even a basic understanding of the intricacies of the brain. Nevertheless, I must ask the fundamental question: Why do normal healthy brain cells stop behaving as they are supposed to behave? What sort of invasion interrupts their natural conformation? Why do they lose contact with their neighborhood? Why do they stop growing and then die in the place where they lived? In particularly vulnerable brain regions – including the amygdale and the hippocampus – what negative initiative interrupts the natural flow of energy – the normal communication between healthy brain cells – that permits aberrant cell to cell behavior? Is it the buildup of abnormally structured plaques between the cells or the intrusion of tangles within affected cells that cause this effect? If these or other physical factors prove to be responsible for the brain's dysfunction, what causes *them* to be out of sync? Are they not atomic entities as well? Our research must broaden to include the abstract spiritual causative factor, the factor that manifests itself as behavior. What causes matter to behave, or not behave?

I have not found any scientific data about the brain and its connection with the mind and the soul. I recently took casual note of a passage in the book *Mayo Clinic on Alzheimer's Disease* regarding the reaction the care giver may experience as he/she cares for a loved one: 'These changes in your relationship and responsibilities can be taxing on your body and soul.'[1] But this use of 'soul' is often used, in a sense, offhandedly in our everyday conversations, so certainly we must not take particular notice of its inclusion in a scientific paper – although we do understand the need to use such a word. However, as what we have deemed to name 'mind' and 'soul' and 'spirit' are not available to hands-on investigation, scientific inquiry has limited access to this sphere of function. The brain can be scanned and examined but its unique capacity to bridge the perceived gap between the physical world and the non-physical world is still unexplored territory. This province is of particular interest to me because I am concerned whether Barbara, stricken with Alzheimer's, is *herself* in harm's way. The outward signs of this debilitating disease are all too apparent, the inability to function in the normal world is obvious, but what about Barbara, her essence, her being, her mind and her soul – is she complete and whole 'inside'?

Alois Alzheimer, a German physician, first diagnosed the disease in 1901. At a scientific meeting in 1906 he introduced the case of a 51 year old woman who had developed memory problems and other symptoms of mental disorder. The condition entered the medical literature a year later when Alzheimer published his findings. In the last century science has discovered much about the brain and these findings are readily available. Current data regarding mental illnesses of all kinds can be accessed through the National Institute of Mental Health's website (http://www.nimh.nih.gov/index.shtml). And we can also keep up to date regarding recent progress in Alzheimer's science and research, thankfully, through services funded by the Alzheimer's Association (http://www.alz.org/index.asp).

Again, it would be unseemly that I, an artist, should attempt to write a paper about Alzheimer's. I have no credentials to validate my point of view. However, I have an obligation to understand, as best I might, the nature of whatever it is that is presented to me. I am not afraid of stepping out of line. I believe there are reasons for everything, even though final answers are most likely closed off to our present level of understanding. But I am wondering about one aspect of the findings in Alzheimer's research that might be misunderstood. The following pages present an argument that I have not found mentioned in the data that has come my way.

The role and power of the non-physical part of us, the part that Energy (capitalized out of respect for its incomprehensibility) plays in facilitating our physical performance, has not been part of the agenda used in scientific research. The possibility that physical matter is more than mere corporeal substance is not even a minor consideration in studying the behavior of atoms, molecules and cells – the constituents of our physical make-up – actually, the components of everything that has a material presence. In general, science has held allegiance to the proposition that answers to perplexing questions about the inner workings of physical matter lie hidden in the recesses of matter itself. This perspective necessarily closes the door to the admission of Energy or 'Spirit' (let us not quibble; it is just a word) as the factor that determines the behavior of things. It is here proposed that so-called physical matter, by itself, is not able to *do* anything. Please bear with me as I attempt to build the foundation for this argument.

Part Four

Questions that Arise

Barbara and I are living our lives in the middle of the most remarkable time of history. Our parents and grandparents (they saw it coming) and our children and grandchildren (they saw it pass) were not quite so favored. The oldest of our lot, my grandfather, was born in 1854 and the youngest, our granddaughter Haley, in 1993. The reason our time is so extraordinary is that an unprecedented surge of scientific discovery has taken place in the span of these few – some 150 – years. We have witnessed a most miraculous transformation. Science tells us that our ancient heritage encompasses Precambrian epochs and that the unnumbered circumstances of life – in essence, the chains and networking of causes and their effects – have brought us to the present day. Certainly 150 years is a mere tick of the evolutionary clock. However, because of this sudden intellectual quickening, the accompanying outpouring of knowledge is changing everything, entirely. I have often wondered: Why wasn't I born perhaps some 500 years ago and why not in some remote Tanganyikan or Peruvian village? And Barbara. How is it that the circumstances of her life should bring us together so that we might find happiness and therewith participate in this sudden fruition of destiny?

Certain questions arise. Studying mankind's history and charting our progress through the tribe, clan and nation, we cannot but ask, 'Is this just a game of chance that we all are here? And, yes, let's include the plants and animals? Are we just thrown together to make a potpourri of sorts, and then, by some remote linkage of happenstance, have the whole business harmonize?' Such serendipity seems unlikely. Every part of a machine is different but for the parts to hum they must be made to correspond. I was talking with an engineer friend who summed it up by saying, 'Everything has to fit.' (He said with his four words what I am attempting to say in 81.)

I wonder about all these things. I'm afraid I'm like the painting, trying to understand what my pigments are made of and who painted me. The task is mine. I am not satisfied or find assurance if I rely on others' convictions and conclusions, even if they are generally acknowledged. But then, am I competent to question such matters? And why, I ask myself, is this so important to me? Why bother?

It is too easy to just sit back and watch the spectacular parade. If I am a part of the whole procession then I matter. And if I matter, then I have a responsibility to do what I should do, and can do, to not be a problem that must be attended to by others, like a squeaky wheel. I must discipline myself to conform to the evolvement in which everything plays its part. I console myself, for I know that countless seekers have asked these same questions, but what if, at this auspicious time, I have more information available than those earlier questioners had? Is there a chance that I might come closer to the mark? I would like to know what is happening to Barbara as she tarries, waiting for Alzheimer's to take her life. Is she secure as her capacities fade away? As her mind becomes clouded and detached, I do not want to pretend that she is not in harm's way. It is an enigma. Alzheimer's and other dementias separate us from this worldly existence without our physical farewell. This is a strange adieu. I see the CAT scan and MRI images. I can see what is happening. But, I remind myself, these are not pictures of Barbara – they are pictures of her brain. Particularly, I would like to know, is science's determination correct, that we are no more than complex organic conglomerations – our atoms and their molecule families merely responding to the music of the spheres, or is this summation, at least in part, wrong? Is there truly a non-physical side of things that is real? Is the mechanistic physical existence all there is to life, or is it, instead, an instrument used to display the spiritual reality within? Are the bodies of plants, animals and people merely costumes that adorn us as we make our way through this terrestrial experience? To be knowable, does Spirit simply clothe itself? I want to know. It is important to me that I know.

The Myth of Materiality

Most of us have a learned fear of getting old and dying. The prospect of consciously stepping into the unknown requires a great deal of courage, especially without some conviction that there is something there to step onto or into. The early explorers needed fortitude to set sail for the horizon, not knowing if they would fall off the world at its edge. We are promised in our holy books that there is a life everlasting waiting, but for the many who do not subscribe to such a doctrine the substantiality of the physical world is very, very convincing. So we go about our business, pledging total allegiance to the materiality of things. What else is there that we can hold onto, all the while getting old, then to find too soon that our grasp is slipping away anyway? Needless to say, signs of aging come our way whether we like it or not. Like unwelcome house guests, they become more wearisome as time goes on. We go to bed at night and the next morning there they are staring at us from our bathroom mirror. They look sort of disheveled, like they didn't sleep well. Maybe it would be a good idea if they moved on.

Well, no, we really don't want to hurry them along. Signs of aging are apparent everywhere. Even the rocks get old. Everything gets older, *except our atoms*. These little guys live forever and never show their age. I asked a doctor friend, 'If my body is made up of eternal atoms and I constantly process their energy, which is always fresh and vibrant, what's getting older?' I don't think he understood my question. I don't think I understood his answer.

Anyway, getting older is a natural attribute of life. As a guileless youngster, I recall thinking I would never get old, certainly not die. 'Life', the word, is difficult to define; it doesn't have any 'substance' to hold onto. We describe it as the 'interval between birth and death'; it is the quality that 'distinguishes living organisms from dead organisms'. This is fine, but where do we go to find dead organisms, or dead anything?

To help explain things, I remind myself of Mr Whipple's fourth grade science class at Haven School where he shared the knowledge that 'Everything is made up of atoms, which cannot be created or destroyed. They can only be transferred from one condition to another.' Apparently this was (and is) more than my mind can grasp, especially when I am told that a drop of water is made up of some 66 billion billion atoms of hydrogen and about 33 billion billion atoms of oxygen! Let's see now: that would mean the oceans, lakes and streams would be made up of, hmm – hmm. And to make things even simpler, Mr Whipple explained that all these atoms are residing contentedly in a stockpile of some 118 elements: iron and carbon and zinc and lithium and such, scattered throughout the cosmos. I do not believe that I am alone. Who can resolve such information? However, in general, science supports Mr Whipple's teaching. Atoms form the substance and structure of every definable form; everything is composed of these miniscule particles. They stand alone. There is no other substance to which they relate. They are the substance.

But then we are faced with another dilemma. Lest we forget, physical matter has no substance. Moving down the scale – bodies and brains to cells to molecules to atoms to nuclei and electrons and protons and neutrons to quarks and electromagnetic fields and pastures – what a fuzzy picture it is. The substance has disappeared. There is nothing there.

And let's take a moment to move up the scale: atoms to molecules to cells and genes to bodies and brains, and then on to metabolism and growth and sense perception and instinct and thought and intellect and ideas and hopes and dreams – what a fuzzy picture *this* is! These tiny bits of matter confuse us. They are, as we say, real, but they are impossible to define. They exist and yet they have no physical presence. They are vibrant but they are passive. For example, these tiny powerful bits of matter do not have a will to *do* anything. They cannot gather themselves to form a rock, flower or animal and thereby facilitate cohesion, growth and sense perception – or for that matter, free will and the capacity to comprehend – human being functions. They cannot foresee their purpose and then stride ahead. Atoms enable thought but they do not think. They are used to facilitate thinking and believing and achieving.

I keep asking myself, 'Is there a way, a perception-path we might uncover that will help us acknowledge the reality of the non-physical realm?' Such a discovery could open whole new worlds of knowledge. With Alzheimer's disease, what prevents certain cells from behaving as they should, that is, the giving birth to new health-building cells? Why are these plaques and tangles able to upset everything? What is, and where lies, the cause of these effects?

Over all, we are addressing the dilemma that the many forms of mental illness impose – striking down unknowable numbers of young and old alike. Referring to the National Institute of Mental Health's statistic, experts estimate '26.2 percent of Americans age 18 and older – about one in four adults – suffer from a diagnosable mental disorder in a given year'. The present paper is not about the symptoms or the progress or the prognosis of these very difficult maladies. We are well informed in these matters. What we do not know is what part of us is hurt and what part of us is not hurt when this tragedy strikes. If we, as researchers, are examining only the physiological aspects of this disease – employing the reliability of analysis and the logic of reason to our scientific inquiry – it is here suggested that this premise may not be inclusive enough. The present agenda does not allow acceptance of the non-physical data that is revealed but is discounted because it is impossible to interpret intellectually. To put aside such evidence is understandable if Energy/Spirit is disproved. However, it is a serious omission if there are evidences of its existence but they are denied merely because of ancient tradition. We cannot afford to disavow that such dysfunction as is evident in Alzheimer's may have, not religious inference but 'spiritual' connotations – whatever this might imply. If such a possibility could be so, an expanded approach to the study and treatment of illnesses of all kinds would be of inestimable value. Life is complex but it is single. Human beings are very complicated but we do know that the two aspects of our being – the physical and the non-physical – intertwine. Regarding the essential oneness of life, the eminent scholar J. E. Esslemont wrote:

> With every advance in science the oneness of the universe and the interdependence of its parts have become more evident. The astronomer's domain is inseparably bound up with the physicist's, and the physicist's with the chemist's, the chemist's with the biologist's, the biologist's with the psychologist's, and so on. Every new discovery in one field of research throws new light on other fields. Just as physical science has shown that every particle of matter in the universe attracts and influences every other particle, no matter how minute or how distant, so psychical science is finding that every soul in the universe affects and influences every other soul.[2]

The key that will open the door to our understanding the mystery of the dual nature of physical matter is itself locked in our interpretation of the findings. Can we review our perception of the workings of life and perchance acknowledge that the *behavior* of all physical forms is other-worldly – but not necessarily closed off to us absolutely?

Partial Information, Lopsided Knowledge

To acknowledge anything, we must touch on its worth, that is, be friendly with its presentation – and then approach a conclusion. At this hour, rational interpretation is our favored tool. Knowledge is based on conclusive evidence, but, still and all, unqualified proofs are elusive. Our understanding is always expanding and thus we are constantly reexamining the evidence shown and revising or strengthening our stand. Early on we thought the world was flat. The premise here stated holds that the knowledge that research has uncovered regarding the workings of life is factual but, in a sense, it has been misinterpreted. There is too much information indicating that there is more happening in the inner workings of physical matter than the mere ongoing display of dancing particles, that when they are behaving themselves, we are sound and whole, and when they are not, we are not. Why are Barbara's brain particles not in step, dancing together?

So where do we go to explore the relationship of the physical and the spiritual aspects of this phenomenon we call life? May I suggest that we follow this path?

Part Five

The Reality of Spirit

The first step that will allow us to acknowledge the reality of the spiritual nature of physical matter is a big step – a leap into unfamiliar territory. We are so accustomed to thinking about ourselves and our surroundings as being real because they are provable through our senses – our eyes and ears and touch and such – that we see no need to look further for proofs or evidences of 'another existence'. In school we were told that our five physical senses unlock the door to knowledge – that if we are missing one or more, our connection to the physical world is significantly diminished. But we were not told that these five tools are bridges that carry information of the physical world to the spiritual world of comprehension, that knowledge of things could lead to the understanding of things. Was it not important to know that eyes look and ears hear and fingers touch and noses smell but we, you and I, we *see*, and we *listen*, and we *feel* and *discern* and *savor*? Eyes do not see; they look; they process light waves so that *we* can attribute meaning to what is being looked at. Why in the world would our teachers want to withhold such information? Was it because it somehow remotely flirted with religious this or that? No wonder our voices hush and our eyes look skyward or askance when some courageous individual in the crowd mentions 'spiritual'.

However, many of the advocates of religious doctrine do not help us with their conclusions either because, for the most part, their summary of things does not incorporate an expanded view of spirituality. With the perspective that is generally current, to be spiritual we must attend church, mosque, synagogue or temple.

Today, in this remarkable period of our history, scientists and researchers and thoughtful thinkers from around the globe are united through their own discoveries and observations and the universal exchange of ideas. As Esslemont stated, every connection and merging brings forth expanded understanding – treasure troves of hidden knowledge in all the fields of their endeavor – enlightenment that was still hidden just a short while ago. The investigation of the spiritual identity of physical matter might well be the next step in the ongoing augmentation of knowledge. Of principal interest to this present discussion is the disclosure that existence is single and that its elemental parts include, without exception, *everything*. Within this verbal template rests the rationale that each and every integral part is vital to the integrity of the whole, and, as well, no part can exist separate and alone; rather there is the stipulation that the smallest, most hidden constituent is as vital as the largest, most obvious one. This entirety includes not only the so-called physical parts of existence but their non-physical counterparts as well, that is, in the reality of what Esslemont and the Mayo Clinic's paper describe as the 'soul'. The miraculous *spiritual behavior* of all the varied *physical* life forms and their overall universal correspondence awakens in us the need to reassess how we are looking at things. Our ocular sight, for example, the one we rely on most, is actually quite unreliable; we see only by way of a very limited wavelength of our sun's total energy.

VISIBLE LIGHT
⇩

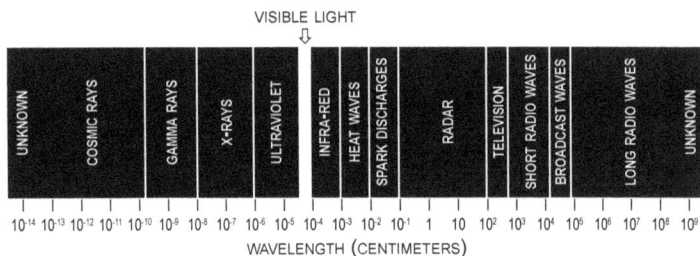

UNKNOWN · COSMIC RAYS · GAMMA RAYS · X-RAYS · ULTRAVIOLET · INFRA-RED · HEAT WAVES · SPARK DISCHARGES · RADAR · TELEVISION · SHORT RADIO WAVES · BROADCAST WAVES · LONG RADIO WAVES · UNKNOWN

10^{-14} 10^{-13} 10^{-12} 10^{-11} 10^{-10} 10^{-9} 10^{-8} 10^{-7} 10^{-6} 10^{-5} 10^{-4} 10^{-3} 10^{-2} 10^{-1} 1 10 10^{2} 10^{3} 10^{4} 10^{5} 10^{6} 10^{7} 10^{8} 10^{9}
WAVELENGTH (CENTIMETERS)

Our terrestrial vision screens most of the 'lights' of the world. How strange our perception of things would be if our eyes were structured just a little differently and we were to make our way with infra-red or gamma sight. Would so subtle a reconfiguration of our atoms and molecules alter our perception of the reality of things?

However, insight, i.e. our inner sight, allows us to *perceive* – to 'see' more than we are focusing on. Such inner vision enables us to investigate reality more inclusively. For instance, all beings, be they mineral, animal, plant or human, though assembled similarly, behave differently, yet their particular integrities correspond and fit together to bring forth a greater perfection than their own. How can it be that the honey bee and the flower correlate unwittingly as they depend absolutely on each other for their existence – and, not incidentally, for ours? Gathered together, we all behave as though we are parts of a single organism. When Barbara was working in the garden up by the road, she became a part of that peaceful setting. The flowers loved her because she was their gardener. They needed her touch, for, left to themselves, they would be overtaken by brambles and thickets. 'Abdu'l-Bahá: '. . . all the members of this endless universe are linked one to another.'[3]

I find it fascinating that behavior, the pivotal factor inherent in the spiritual world, becomes apparent only through the agency of the physical world. For example, let us consider the forest pond as a universe. On close examination, atoms abound everywhere. Each drop of water, every lily pad and pollywog, similarly composed, comprise the whole. They interact, behave, without will, perfectly – perform as a single organism, naturally. However, although their different outer structures are marvelously adapted to their surrounding environment, it is not their different shapes and sizes that are vital to the life of the pond – these are merely expedient configurations of atoms. It is their inner spiritual capacities that correspond and enhance one another to enable the existence of their micro universe. Spiritual behavior – represented in the pond as cohesion and growth and sense perception – is the featured performer hidden in this forest setting. These attributes are life's attributes, and they are spiritual, that is, non-physical, in that they do not have a material aspect. Evidences of the reality of Energy/Spirit are apparent everywhere, not only in the forest pond. Reading Esslemont's commentary again, compatibility, the natural affinity of being to being, is a spiritual condition. If a living system functions with conformity, balance and order are maintained. Teilhard de Chardin championed the truth when he wrote:

> Love alone is capable of uniting living beings in such a way as to complete and fulfill them, for it alone takes them and joins them by what is deepest in themselves.
>
> Considered in its full biological reality, love – that is to say, the affinity of being with being – is not peculiar to man. It is a general property of all life and as such it embraces, in all its varieties and degrees, all the forms successfully adapted by organized matter . . . And in fact if we look around us at the confluent ascent of consciousness, we see it is not lacking anywhere.[4]

This unity of purpose is essential to the function of life. If some fragment of the 'whole' steps out of line, every other component is affected. This has been affirmed in the study of the connections between the cells of the brain. If there is an imbalance in the organization of the integral parts of the brain, there will be a universal consequence: 'every soul in the universe affects and influences every other soul'.[5] Unity and harmony evoke affinity and accord; the lack of unity appears as incompatibility and disassociation. The spiritual aspect of life is indeed a powerful force.

How this spiritual force manifests itself is intriguing. A few evenings ago I was having supper with Barbara, and Don was seated at our table. He suddenly dropped his fork and pressed his hands to his head and cried out, 'Oh! The pain, the pain.' I immediately called to a care manager and she hurriedly summoned a nurse. I tried to console him, assuring him that help was on the way, and Barbara reached over and gently placed her hand on his arm and lovingly said – without any fumbling for words – 'The nurse is coming, and she is very pretty.' Barbie has not been able to coherently put words together for months. What was it that enabled the tangled connections in her brain to facilitate this extraordinary behavior? What 'force' enabled her to do this?

What is it that transpires when we look into the eyes of a loved one? What transfers through the hand to the heart when a strong grasp (or a limp one) is returned? The bearing, the relevance of the spiritual force that motivates the physical world must be embraced and called upon when addressing dysfunctional and debilitating behavior. Its reality is apparent in all of our modes – when we are happy or sad, contemplative or light-hearted. This will be a new venture; there is little data that supports conclusively the validity of spiritual healing. The laying of strong hands on a weak body is known to be beneficial. The tenor and tone of soothing words – in all, the presence and strength of Energy/Spirit, however manifested, connect the strong with the weak in miraculous ways. This force is single but it is constantly being cycled and recycled appropriately throughout creation. There is no reason to suggest that we cannot willfully take part in its dissemination.

As was stated earlier, in the midst of this momentous flood of knowledge that we are witnessing today, of marked interest because they affect us so personally, are the achievements in the field of medical science. Technology has dramatically broadened our knowledge of the workings of the mechanistic world – the world of thermodynamics and nuclear physics. As our researchers delve deeper and deeper, a slight misstep could alert a particularly receptive mind and point us in a different dimension so that we might see more clearly the spiritual nature of the physical matter that is being examined. Perhaps we are in need of a contemporary René Descartes who will, with wonder, look up from his experiments and proclaim, 'Yes, yes! I see. Now I see!' With anticipation we look to an expanded field of inquiry to explore the true nature of the physical world

– why it acts as it does – and, along the way, find a more holistic treatment and cure for many mental afflictions, certainly including clinical depression and schizophrenia as well as Alzheimer's. And who knows whether then the dysfunction caused by cancer and Parkinson's and diabetes might be more comprehensively addressed? At this juncture, we activists must be courageous and ask ourselves, 'What if, by chance or design, there actually *is* another world waiting for the investigative unbiased mind, a counterpart non-physical world, the attributes of which will be easily recognized and defined as opposites of those of the physical one?' Counterbalances are essential; one condition without the other is meaningless. (A straight line is unknowable without our knowing a crooked one; an open door itself defines the closed one.) The frailties of mind and body would be unknowable were it not for sound health and strong will. The material world, through its own presence, demands a non-physical counterpart. When the scientist insists that only the material world exists, we cannot but ask what is the other factor that gives the material world its acknowledged identity? What might we name what it is that the physical world is not? Metaphysical? No? Well, so be it, but let's give it a definitive name. Spirit/Energy will do. Perhaps, for this assignment, our agenda should be based on the assumption that 'the spiritual' exists, and then set out to disprove the premise. As pioneers, we remind ourselves that, in our search for truth, our credo stipulates that no avenue to knowledge can be closed off to us.

Strangely, the existence of the spiritual world is revealed to us each and every day – from the moment we are born. Using our miraculous physical senses – seeing, hearing, touching, etc. – we are constantly connecting to the world of meaningful abstraction. As stated earlier, our eyes look but we process the observed data and enhance it with meaning. Throughout our lifetime we use the information gathered through our senses, and as we grow older, we not only mature physically but spiritually as well. Our senses can reveal the hidden, deeper meaning tying knowledge of things to their significance. They serve to reveal the spiritual aspect of our humanity. Erich Fromm:[6]

> Physical birth, if we think of the individual, is by no means as decisive and singular an act as it appears to be. . . Actually, the process of birth continues. The child learns to speak, it learns to know the function of things; it learns to relate itself to others, to avoid punishment and gain praise and liking. Slowly, the growing person learns to love, to develop reason, to look at the world objectively. He begins to develop his powers; to acquire a sense of identity, to overcome the seduction of his senses for the sake of an integrated life. Birth, then, in the conventional meaning of the word, is only the beginning of birth in the broader sense. The whole life of the individual is nothing but the process of giving birth to himself: indeed, we should be fully born when we die . . .[7]

Though it is not for me to say, I do believe that Barbara was fully born when Alzheimer's shortened her life. Even though she could not communicate her concerns and feelings as the later stages of this disease assumed command, she was able to teach all who were close to her and knew her about life's greatest lesson, the guidance that enables us to be happy in all circumstances: that is, to be radiantly acquiescent, no matter what.

As these later stages gained control over Barbara's life, she maintained her determination to carry on. At this moment, seated at my computer, writing her story, I am wearing one of the sweaters she made for me. It is much too large but I love it. Towards the last years she had difficulty counting the stitches and following the instructions and now, looking back, I wonder how many times we went to the Yarn Basket to have her efforts pulled apart and the pattern restored, and how many times I went to the print shop to have the directions made larger. But this was not the problem. Alzheimer's was the problem.

Part Six

Disclosures

If we were asked to describe the networking that defines our human condition, most likely many of us would fumble around to find the right words and then struggle to put them into sequence; such considerations are not ordinary ones. We are physical and we are non-physical. It's easy to identify our physical realness because it's right here facing us in our mirror and toting us around. But our other parts and their relationships are a bit vague. Some long years ago I found the explanations of 'Abdu'l-Bahá[8] satisfying because they stand to reason and extraordinary because they are to the point. I will paraphrase but, of course, it would be best to refer to the original texts.[9]

The *brain* is the physical instrument of the mind. The *mind* is the non-physical instrument of the soul and is used to fathom the mysteries – the deeper meanings hidden in the appearance of things – thereby enabling the soul to develop. The *human soul* is the individualized expression of spirit, i.e. spirit manifested in the human degree. *Spirit* itself is the wondrous, indestructible, indivisible energy infusing life in all of existence. And of course the *body* – the brain included – is the physical instrument that facilitates, in this setting, the soul's development and growth.

These words, like all words, have been invented to serve a particular need. That science may not like some of them is understandable if their why and wherefore is superfluous, not needed, that is, if these non-physical states of being do not exist. But as there is indisputable evidence that they do exist, we have to name them something, so let's go along with mind, soul and spirit – they are just words.

'Abdu'l-Bahá's clarification of the relationship of our essential non-physical parts leads us to conclude that the brain is not the storehouse where thought and memory abide but is rather the apparatus that processes information for the soul's advantage and use. This would mean that the brain *does not* hold information but only accesses it. The Mayo Clinic paper on Alzheimer's states that 'almost every part of the brain is involved in memory storage'.[10] Apparently this is a general consensus, for this summary is the unwavering answer to my question at book reviews and seminars. When I pose the question, experts respond similarly. However, I cannot posit that the brain is the repository for knowledge but I can understand that its function is to be receptive to knowledge, and I can understand that the brain is equipped to consign it and access it. These are mechanistic functions. As the body of knowledge processed by the brain is non-physical, its rightful home must be in the spiritual domain. Referring again to the relationship of our parts, it becomes clear that the soul, through the power of the mind, is the repository for memory. With this premise we then can understand that the factual data, collected through our five-sense perception, is, in a manner of speaking, 'food' for the soul wherein it is processed into meaning; and there it will abide until our free will calls it forth – through the capacities of the mind and the instrument of the brain.[11] As this cognitive 'material' is without a physical aspect, then its storeroom is not in the physical brain but in the spiritual domain. *But* this is a logical conclusion only if such a domain is granted. Science is still hesitant to acknowledge the existence of the distinct mind and soul, and thus admit to such a networking of 'unproven' human attributes. However, such conjecture is called upon when we question what it is that happens when inspired thoughts – thoughts that have no prior existence and thus cannot be drawn from a warehouse of existing knowledge stored in our brain cells – emerge. We dream of eventualities yet to come and we find answers to questions unanswerable in our waking hours – all appearing *through* the instrument of the brain – their origin obviously coming from 'outside'.

Barbara's ability to console Don when he was in pain could be facilitated by her brain cells, in this particular instance, networking differently – linking heretofore unrelated cells to enable fine-tuned expressiveness in the configuration of words stored in her soul. Oftentimes clear thought is inexplicably channeled through tangled cells in an Alzheimer's afflicted brain. Barbara's surprising comment, 'The nurse is coming' was a repeat of my words to Don but 'and she is very pretty' were her words, and certainly they were not stored as such and intact in the cells of her brain because the entire event had just happened. She was drawing on the natural sensitivities of her earlier life. *This is very significant.* If this is the case, it would mean that the mind, the tool of the soul, the essence of one's being, is not affected aversely when Alzheimer's or other dementias intervene and impair the brain. This quotation from 'Abdu'l-Bahá explains further:

> Some think that the body is the substance and exists by itself, and that the spirit is accidental and depends upon the substance of the body, although, on the contrary, the rational soul is the substance, and the body depends upon it. If the accident – that is to say, the body – be destroyed, the substance, the spirit, remains.
>
> Second, the rational soul, meaning the human spirit, does not descend into the body – that is to say, it does not enter it, for descent and entrance are characteristics of bodies, and the rational soul is exempt from this. The spirit never entered this body, so in quitting it, it will not be in need of an abiding-place: no, the spirit is connected with the body, as this light is with this mirror. When the mirror is clear and perfect, the light of the lamp will be apparent in it, and when the mirror becomes covered with dust or breaks, the light will disappear.[12]

I interpret this to mean that the body and brain are parts of our physical make-up and thus they are subject to the laws of nature but the soul and its instrument the mind are spiritual entities that are not acted upon or altered by the limitations of the material world. The mind is the median that connects the brain with the human spirit. This is a new way of looking at things. Living matter, body and brain included, is relegated to the station of servitude.

All of the above supports the premise that physical substance is the matrix Spirit uses for its own purpose and that alone matter is without intrinsic worth. Thus when the plant, animal or human being 'dies', its assembled particles are recycled and they then unwittingly participate in another cause, but the Energy that used these particles remains unaffected, intact. This Energy, locked in the atom, is powerful beyond measure. (We fear the day when it will destroy us all.) Each and every form so engaged necessarily places restrictions on Energy's fuller emanation. The rock allows a particular degree (cohesion); the plant a greater measure (growth) and the animal permits even more (instinct and sense perception). We human beings, embracing the capacities of the 'lesser beings', show forth Energy/Spirit in ever greater intensity with the powers of the mind (intellect and reason).

Although it is true that I have no academic credentials to validate my stand regarding the connection of the brain and the mind, I do have the freedom to consider – without bias – all possibilities that are presented. I am not shackled by age-old perceptions that perhaps stifle a new-world outlook. 'Abdu'l-Bahá has the necessary credentials and His insightful perspective opens up a vision of the oneness of reality – the reality that we call life – that heretofore has been closed off to us. I have found no other hypothesis that addresses this course of study. Throughout former ages knowledge followed a progressive path. By way of logical argument and reasonable consideration, understanding has increasingly enhanced human perceptivity. Now the reality of Spirit and its influence in the material world is made clearer. 'Abdu'l-Bahá takes the material world and hands it to us on a spiritual platter.

What our true state is when our minds can no longer be accessed is unknowable. Even when we are mentally keen, we live in the world of limited perception, unconscious of our essential well-being. How far would we have to go to strip away the material non-essentials – to then find our unadorned spiritual selves? As our lives unfold, we are concerned that we have mattered. Going through the daily routines – all the while getting old – hardly seems worthwhile unless there are assurances of an ultimate meaning hidden within us. The premise of this essay is that the essence of life resides in the spiritual world and that the material world is an illusion. The essential part of all life forms – minerals, plants, animals and human beings – is their essence, that is, their non-physical/spiritual attributes, the attributes that give them their identity and, not incidentally, facilitate the world's behavior – every aspect of the world's behavior.

In the human realm individuality plays a vital role, for each of us has particular capacities and capabilities. These attributes are obviously not of our choosing. We can have no concept of what particular need our lives might satisfy in the furtherance of life's plan. All we can know is that life's workings are very economical; similar to the forest pond, there isn't any waste. Though we cannot appraise our personal worth and place it appropriately in the scheme of things, we must assume that every integral part of a natural system is vital to its function. However, we cannot know if the imposition of physical restraints absolutely shields the radiance of our spiritual influence. Can we know the source of an idea? Where is the repository where hope and courage and love reside?

Thus, Spirit is the reality. Henceforth, we must acknowledge that our residence is in the spiritual world and then balance our factual knowledge to comply with the spiritual laws that define behavior. We must find the holistic approach that will allow us to address life's dual nature. It will be a joyful celebration. Until then, we can have the assurance that Alzheimer's does not, in any way, harm us.

Watching Barbara while I was tending to her needs was like going to school again. Apparently I am not too old to learn.

She taught me that she was being cleansed of the world. From the world's viewpoint this was bad; from her spirit's perspective this was good.

INTERMISSION

*Scientific investigation does not lead to knowledge
of the intrinsic nature of things.*
Sir Arthur Eddington

Part Seven

A New Perspective: Resolutions

The Premise

It is proposed that a heritage and lifetime of passive thinking is a contributing factor to the susceptibility of Alzheimer's appearance in one's later life. The management of routine circumstances that are presented through the course of the day – day after day after day – will make real the mind's capacity to react solely to happenings. Its ability to facilitate vigorous initiative and creative thinking will be left unattended.

The Analogy

Teaching children to process information that comes exclusively from outside the province of their own origination has far-reaching consequences. With this stoic agenda the children will know only what their books tell them and they will not know what constitutes their individual worth. Today children are conditioned to memorize and remember volumes of information, endless pages of facts and figures. They are programmed to store this knowledge and, when the test day comes, call forth certain fragments and fill in the blank spaces with appropriate answers. If they manage this task well, they will be moved on to the next grading level and repeat the process. The end product will be a diploma and supper at the Pancake House. The children's essential capacities will be neglected.

The magnitude, complexity and fine-tuning of the machinery that produces so meager an output are daunting. Elaborate structures and equipment are continually being upgraded. Yet the classroom is an austere center, generally not considered an exciting place to discover yearning, interests and understanding. Not so long ago, the purpose of the educational system was to prepare children for a practical life. However, as the years passed, more and more information was made available and more and more children were gathered together to learn. Today the gatherings are too large and there is too much information to remember. Learning by rote circumvents the children's need to understand the *significance* of what they are studying. Thus their thinking is impaired – and their teachers are forthwith indefensibly frowned upon with disapproval. The dysfunction lies elsewhere.

At this hour the purpose of schooling should be to teach children to think. If they can only remember things, their knowledge is shallow and their minds are left crippled. When it comes time to credit all the lessons with meaning – to connect with abstract thought and therewith bring forth personal, particular, expressive and meaningful ideas – they are lost. The view that the brain's purpose is merely to stockpile information is a very conservative evaluation of the potential that lies in its astounding structure. Ascribing to the brain a purely utilitarian function, where information is stowed away in the memory bank and then called upon when needed, does not allow for the creative factor, which is its primary and phenomenal sphere of function. The point is made: Without our comprehending the essential province of the brain, the children's propensity for mental acuity will not be addressed and they will merely grow old. This is the analogy.

Brain, the Tool of the Mind

The human brain is alive, a living organism. When Energy is able to use the constituent parts of the brain in normal ways, the owner of this system will be able to function and behave naturally – natural for that individual. Thus the living brain becomes the instrument that allows individuality and personality to be displayed. These attributes, in themselves, do not have a physical presence; they are illusive, non-physical qualities that serve to represent and define a particular human being. We must assume that these qualities are given a venue through the wondrous material composition that is formulated at conception. Individual distinctness comes into being when the components of egg and sperm meet. These 'particles' are infused with a genetic heritage that will accompany the individual throughout his/her life. Martha Graham:[13]

> There is a vitality, a life force, an energy, a quickening that is translated through you into action, and because there is only one of you in all of time, this expression is unique. And if you block it, it will never exist through any other medium and it will be lost. The world will not have it. It is not your business to determine how good it is nor how valuable nor how it compares with other expressions. It is your business to keep it yours clearly and directly, to keep the channel open.[14]

In order to contemplate the structure of the brain, science has had to invent a unique vocabulary to designate the cerebral parts and their relationships. The basic constituents are, of course, atoms, atoms of elements that are combined in a particular manner and measure. The atoms' interplay, their chemistry, the way they are assembled and the way they pair off and hook up, require a sophisticated nomenclature. RIBONUCLEIC ACID, the double helix structure of DEOXYRIBONUCLEIC ACID, genes and genomes and exons and introns are necessary to describe the inner structure of cerebral matter but these words essentially describe only the physical machinery that enables the spiritual performance; actually, the effect is more remarkable than the cause. The terrestrially formed brain, atoms selected from the warehouse of 118 known elements, miraculously authorizes intellectual perception – *but only if it is invigorated*.

Although the cause of Alzheimer's is still open to question, early testing through MRI scanning suggests that a forthcoming diagnosis can be made even decades before the symptoms appear. Images of the progressive shrinkage of the hippocampus, a region of the brain that shows some of the first signs of Alzheimer's disease long before the condition spreads to the cerebral cortex and results in cognitive and memory impairment, foretell what the future holds. After death the plaques and tangles and disclosed dead cells will confirm the diagnosis. But when brain tissue is examined under the microscope, the observer is not examining the brain; he or she is looking at cerebral matter – enlarged images of cells that were once used by the living brain, physical structures that in their former state allowed brain behavior. Now they allow only atomic and molecular behavior, very humble and constrained allowances. Is it really possible that such base matter can interpret the 'secret' that at one time used it for its habitation? To anticipate finding the mystery of the living tree in the fallen leaf is most likely a vain hope.

As the value of the brain lies in its function, our appraisal of its merit necessarily must focus on its behavior when it is alive. What sustains the brain and what harms the brain should be our main concern. If its strength and well-being somehow necessitate intellectual stimuli, then the dull and dreary diet of factual knowledge will not be satisfying and will eventually lead to starvation. This deprivation is particularly of the mind, but we might assume the brain, its tool, languishes as well: to function in the material world, their capacities are necessarily connected and reciprocal. The networking is described above on pages 51 to 54.

Today, the magnitude and complexity of the information presented for our consideration – to children and adults alike – are overwhelming. Superficialities screen the verities of life. We are, in a sense, martyrs of our time, having to 'surrender' so much to find anything of real value. Not so long ago, primary education focused its attention on teaching letters and numbers and a smattering of facts because this agenda was quite sufficient to prepare us for work on the farm and in the factory. Just a generation or two ago there wasn't the need to revitalize this system of instruction in order to adapt to dramatic intellectual stimulus. Tending the store or working the fields did not require creative thought – only knowledge was needed so that the inventory could be kept up and plantings might be sown in accord with the seasons. Schools did not prepare us to be creative in the processing of ideas because outside the classroom there was no need to foster a dream in a quiescent world.

When Barbara and I moved to this assisted care center, most of the residents here at the time had grown up with this basic schoolroom training – remembering information so that they could get a diploma and find work. This was made clear one morning after our exercise class. Kim, our Activities Coordinator, suggested we speak about our dreams – thoughts we had when we were young. It went something like this:

Kim: 'Let's tell about our dreams. Not sleepy dreams but dreams that we had when we were little. Edith, what were your dreams?'

Edith: 'Well, let's see. Hmm, well, I went to school and I grew up and worked at the bank. And . . . ah, hmm . . . I got married and had two children, well, that's about it. Oh, I also went to church. Dreams. No, I don't think I had any dreams. No, I just worked at the bank.'

Kim: 'Ruth, what were your dreams?'

Around the circle the question went, and the only difference in the responses was that the bank turned into the dry goods store or the post office or the grocery. Most of those present had symptoms of Alzheimer's disease.

I remember my mother's comment. She must have said it more that once because I can still see the picture so clearly in my mind's eye. Relaxing together in our living room after supper, friends – and dad – would be enthusiastically talking and mother would be sitting 'over there' quietly knitting.

When the conversations turned to speculations and ideas and deeper meanings, mom would look up and say whimsically, 'You're going to wear your brains out.' Mother in her late years had Parkinson's and symptoms of dementia. Her death certificate is inscribed 'brain disease'.

My dear Barbara, too, did not like to talk about ideas. Like my mother, amidst all her wonderful qualities, she shied away from abstract thought. Now, when I have supper with her in her dining room, waiting for the meal to be served, she will fold and unfold her napkin, in a sense symbolically practicing what she did in the daily routines of her earlier life. But if I try to balance a spoon on its side, she will immediately knock it over and brush it away. If I arrange some jelly beans in a row or sort them by color, Barbara will not recognize the pattern or 'see' any meaning. Although she is suffering from the advanced stages of Alzheimer's, traces of her earlier pattern of behavior still make their presence known.

Because Alzheimer's is today so common an affliction, I am suggesting that there is a connection between the passive mind set of an unchallenging intellectual lifestyle – so characteristic of former times – and the sudden demands imposed on our reasoning faculties today. I am proposing that minds without stimulus become passionless and indifferent. With the present surge of information and the deluge of challenging circumstances that require cognition and appraisal and resolution – conditions necessarily calling on the employment of creative thought – minds retreat, having been programmed to maintain the status quo for so long. They thus become, in a sense, less vital, even traumatized. Under the sudden onset and onslaught of unprecedented cerebral challenge, rather than to enter the fray and adapt to the progress, their capacities lie dormant. And even more: As the world outside moves on, these zestless reasoning faculties regress in that they are increasingly distanced from the ongoing escalation. I remember that when our children left for college Barbara lost more of her initiative; their sudden departure left a void that could not be replaced with anything, not even a hobby. I wonder if this hollow, and other subtle but salient changes along the way, could have left her vulnerable to Alzheimer's. Now, it is quite apparent; when something unfamiliar happens, or a change of any kind presents itself, Barbara will retreat, withdraw, and this divorce will leave its mark unless it is very temporary, in which case she will appear to forget that it happened. If it is permanent, like our move from the country to the city, the effect will be lasting. A different and more isolating norm will embrace and hold her.

We all shy away from change; it is characteristic of people. Perhaps the repetitiousness of the daily routine, the waking and working, the repeat of the seasons – and all the rest – condition us to seek security in keeping things as they are. However, we know that change is inevitable; nothing stays the same. Getting older, for instance, is such a gradual transformation that it is hardly noticed – until suddenly we find we are blowing out an additional candle on the cake. Subtle change is acceptable, but, if it is too out of the ordinary, it swallows us up. The changes that are taking place at this auspicious time in our cultural and societal and technological evolvement are unprecedented. Never before have we had to mentally adjust to transitions introduced so unexpectedly and suddenly. The Industrial Revolution brought changes that were previously inconceivable. We accepted some of the new bestowals with gratitude – Jonas Salk's vaccine eliminated the scourge of poliomyelitis, and how thankful we are – and with alacrity, as in 1920 when the first radio station opened up in Pittsburg and everyone crowded around to listen to anything that came across the waves. Television shook us up a bit but we gave in. However, just a few years later when the word processing computer and Internet entered the scene, these very same people thought that this was too big a jump from the comfortable, manageable typewriter and telephone and they let this kind of technology pass. It came on too quickly; the whole proposition was too different to contemplate. It is hard to realize that as an artless youngster I played with a radio wave crystal set. Over the span of a single generation, the refinement of technology and the opening of the floodgate of knowledge left many of us behind – alone and at rest in a quiet solitude. I am proposing that this tranquil state renders the mind and its servant brain defenseless against the unfamiliar and sudden imposition of abstract thought.

The Passive Brain

We might say the mind is the master and the brain its machine but we are on shaky ground when we take a stand and talk about the brain's sphere of function. In answer to my question at seminars, the brain and the mind are often placed under the same canopy, the one analogous to the other, perhaps similar in function but not in structure. For the most part, we like to talk about the physical brain but we haven't much patience with matters of the distinct mind because many of us are still not able to acknowledge that there is more grandeur and transcendental worth to the brain than the intricate alignment of its particles. The uncomfortable alliance, which serves to connect the physical brain to a particular pattern of spiritual performance, is a mystery that complicates current research because there are not enough hard facts to work with that might lead to such affirmation, that is, that the brain is physical and the mind is not. However, such a word as 'networking' – the networking of the brain cells – is readily acknowledged. With a microscopic cant to this word's meaning we will understand that networking describes a societal condition that allows impartial, uncommitted cells to have relationships. The resultant organization defines the environment wherein the cells live and grow and communicate, and this nurturing setting does not have a material aspect. What this environment does is enable communal 'behavior' and this attribute is illusive to scrutiny. However, in the case of Alzheimer's disease, what we are dealing with is the uncooperative mutual relationship of the brain cells and not just their physical structure. I suspect that brain cells are not generic, that they are not neutral entities that have no particular formulation, but rather that they carry our personal imprint, or at least the imprint of a particular evolutionary moment. Is today's brain cell disposition, like the child grown old, the end product of prior formative eras, which up to the present has been accustomed to behave in only a perfunctory way? Pragmatically, are these cells transferable from one brain to another and, if so, would a theoretical sampling of a pre-Neolithic brain – a brain occupied with the most fundamental and mundane of concerns – be adaptable to a contemporary one, one assailed by stimulating propositions as never before? Could the brain/mind's lackadaisical heritage incline it to brushing aside the need to adjust rapidly to the obligation, the necessity and challenge of intellectual stimulation which is the criterion of our time?

I am proposing that the minds of many of today's Alzheimer's victims take on a passivity characterized by the habit of merely processing information that comes along. Thus they are unready to respond to challenging intellection and to adapt to the unforeseeable imposition of intellectual acuity, characterized today by the necessity of lifting knowledge to the realm of understanding; that is, to the management and refinement of ideas. There may even be a carryover into our son's generation: he reports that few of his professional associates have thoughts to share. These individuals are very competent at their jobs but it would seem they are uncomfortable with considerations that touch on abstract out-of-the-office ideas or meaningful reflection. They work, come home to be with the family, fix the fence or play golf but that's about it. It is not that they are not mentally keen, for their knowledge and expertise are most likely exemplary. It rests, rather, in the exercise of the mind, through the capacities of the brain to the degree that knowledge is put to use for abstract thought – meditative, evocative thought. This is the premise for this essay. Obviously there are many individuals who may be passive in the exercising of their minds but who are not taken down by Alzheimer's disease; and there are undoubtedly many who are extraordinarily creative whose lives are cut short by this plague, but the fact remains that Alzheimer's is unexplainably gaining ground and to this date running rampant. If we find the answer with our scanners and scopes, good! But so far we are able to look only at the appearance of things. Spirit is passed over.

If it is plausible that Alzheimer's is more apt to find residence in a brain that has been passive through most of its life, then we must better prepare oncoming generations to find in their inner selves the seeds of a purposefully vibrant life so that they may prosper mentally in correspondence with the demands of the expanding world. We must be vigilant in helping our children realize their essential worth. They must become independent thinkers, responsible for their decisions and not blindly, lackadaisically follow others' lead, others who need them to strengthen their own agendas. This would mean that they must gradually prepare themselves to question every premise and every proposition, certainly including postulates in the fields of religion, science, education and government. They must have strong, unwavering personal aspirations and set goals attuned to their time. Then the changes that are taking place throughout the world will be more readily managed and assimilated by minds prepared for edification and change.

The reason that current scientific inquiry may not be able to focus on the cause and cure of Alzheimer's and other dementias is that physical matter is much more than it appears to be. Physical substance is an enabling agent, a go-between that connects universal Energy with particularized behavior – the manner and mode in which living beings function. For example, a particular assortment of atoms and molecules, when aligned in a particular way, will bring forth a certain mineral, a special flower, a specific animal or a unique and beautiful child. Whatever form physical matter assumes, it behaves as its composition allows; its form is determined by its function. If the integral parts, the atoms and molecules, are arranged in compatible ways, the system will perform normally and there will be no excess. If the alignment of the integral parts is not compatible, there will be dysfunction – and waste, as in the case of Alzheimer's disease, where the brain's natural and normal configuration is corrupted with invasive plaques and tangles and there are dead leavings that serve no purpose. In a healthy, vibrant brain, each atom, molecule and cell is necessary to sustain its equilibrium, and there is no residue.

The Vibrant Brain

My premise is that the spiritual nature of physical matter has not yet been recognized. If this is the case, then the contemporary brain can be made responsive and functional through the expanded activity of the mind. Rather than being sedentary, at ease, casually processing information as it comes into range, it becomes quickened, keen – full of Energy! It is here proposed that this vitality will be brought about by expanding the mind's capacity to reason and to comprehend. The brain's intended function will be nurtured and brought to life through the consciousness, learning, proficiency, scholarship, erudition and perseverance of the mind.

I suggest that fortifying the mind will enable it to better deal with the effects of the Alzheimer's gene or will hinder or prevent it from taking effect. It is here proposed that the aggressive, inhospitable Alzheimer gene will not then be able to reign over its former passive, now energized neighbors. Genes are merely genes; they are neither good nor bad until they exert their influence in the community. If they are out of sync with their environment, they are labeled 'bad'. Concentrating on the bad gene and rendering it feeble is one way to address the problem. But what if this approach is not feasible or even possible? If we are dealing with the non-physical behavior of physical matter – which is what I am suggesting – customary inquiry and sophisticated but ordinary remedial procedures may not be relevant. If not, the resolution might be found in the other of our two realms, the domain where non-physical realities prosper, where balance and compatibility and conformity naturally allow life to advance. To achieve this, it is here suggested that we must alert the mind, strengthen it with initiative, infuse it with vitality and energize it with confidence. These attributes do not have a physical presence but they do exist. Rather than concentrating on attacking the 'bad' cells or genes to make them weaker, we concentrate on making the weak 'good' cells stronger – giving them muscle through charging their cerebral environment with Energy. Their configuration and well-being will then comply with their prescribed and current capability. Then Alzheimer's disease, the brain's dreaded opponent, will fade away naturally as there will be no slumbering, quiet place for it to incubate and grow.

We must start with our children. We must find an agenda that will foster their dreams and nurture their souls, an agenda that will alert them to the requisites of their time in history and instill in their consciousness assurances of their competency. They must be taught to weigh every proposition that comes their way and learn from its influence. They must enter the garden of human diversity with all the individuality that they possess – with all that they have been given – and be vital and significant. They must be taught to be searchers after truth.[15]

Our time is a privileged time. We are, at last, seeing the light at the end of the tunnel through which humanity has long groped its way. As we emerge from the darkness, we will use all that we have learned in the past and will, with wonder, uncover basic knowledge to reveal unimaginable insight and understanding. All thinking will reflect the new vitality; the expansion of the mind will disclose answers that heretofore were unanswerable. This dawning will light the path to the future and it will reveal a core oneness to which everything must conform. Incompatibilities such as Alzheimer's disease will fall victim to this revolution and be heard of no more.

Part Eight

Barbara's Passing

As Barbara's illness progressed, she increasingly appeared to be in a world apart, one that I could not share with her or even comprehend. Now I understand better. When Barbara asked about her mother and her sister – 'Have you heard from mom? And Mary Ellen, did she call?' – she was not bringing them back from the past but was looking for them in her present, anticipating their companionship. It gradually dawned on me that Barbara was already significantly, predominantly in the spiritual world. What I interpreted to be her departure was instead a gradual arrival at the shore of the realm beyond. She had already moved on. This adieu started long before her physical passing, and, as the months turned into years, she returned to me only fleetingly and on special occasions. She became innocent and childlike. Early on, she would look at me and identify me with, 'You're Harlan.' But later, looking puzzled, she would ask, 'You're Harlan?' She was tied to me spiritually, and my physical appearance – ever older and more wrinkled – confused her. 'Where is the one I married?' 'Who is this old guy?' I now realize that Barbara knew me *only by way of my spiritual attributes*, and the corporeal costume I was wearing was distracting. My image and my words and my world now held no meaning for her. When I touched the spoon to her lips there was little response. Alzheimer's had taken this world from her and she was left pure and unburdened.

Now I more fully grasp, through her ingenuousness, that this material world truly is an illusion, that the real world is hidden behind the appearance of things. Barbara helped me understand that, from the start of our relationship, we had found the mutual attraction that naturally bonds life to a purpose – to its purpose. Barbara and I shared the affinity that is infused in all life's forms. Through her teaching I learned that this spiritual attraction transcends the physical; that we become one with the lesser creatures and the universe itself – as soul mates; that we are spiritual beings at the moment of our physical conception.

When Barbara was ready to pass on, lying in the hospital bed barely breathing, barely here, she was powerfully intentioned. Willfully holding her atoms and molecules sufficiently intact, she waited the necessary hours for her family to gather from distant locations to be at her side. Then she breathed a sigh in acknowledgment and let loose. As we quietly looked upon her countenance, our daughter Nancy was moved to say, 'It's a picture of Mom.'

Note

This essay is, in a sense, the consequence of an intrigue, a natural corollary to a lifetime love affair with the ideas and interpretations of the renowned 'Abdu'l-Bahá. I have found His explanations regarding the nature of the physical world, the duality of its presentation and the unity that is inherent therein, fundamental and profound. However, these teachings became even more relevant to my life when Barbara's illness was diagnosed as Alzheimer's disease.

In a very real sense, Barbara was my qualified teacher. As I endeavored to care for her, I also watched her carefully as the months turned into years, until her passing on December 10, 2008. I took notes as her illness progressed and these observations gradually evolved into this treatise.

In the beginning, I did not anticipate that these teachings would be pertinent to Barbara's mental disorder. Nor was I aware that 'Abdu'l-Bahá's explanations concerning the relationship of the brain, mind, soul and spirit, expounded almost a century ago, might be pertinent to human perceptivity only at this time. These are not my ideas. However, that His elucidations, Barbara's illness and the present need for answers to the Alzheimer's dilemma should coincide is, I believe, ordained – as fanciful as this might seem.

The acknowledgment of Spirit as the pith and substance of all matter will change everything. We all are path finders and bridge builders, taking part in the evolution of human destiny, and there are milestones that mark our progress. At one time we were gatherers and hunters preparing the way for explorers and researchers, all the while becoming acquainted with the physical world that we found to be our habitat. We did not choose our time but we did serve to bring forth ever greater manifestations of life's purpose; that is; the refinement of matter to reveal the fuller reflection of Spirit. Now, apparently, we are ready to intellectually explore this non-physical reality, the reality that lies hidden behind the appearance of things.

Bibliography

'Abdu'l-Bahá. *Selections from the Writings of 'Abdu'l-Bahá*. Haifa: Bahá'í World Centre, 1978.

— *Some Answered Questions*. Wilmette, IL: Bahá'í Publishing Trust, 1981.

— Tablet to August Forel. *Bahá'í World*, vol. 15. Haifa: Bahá'í World Centre, 1976, pp. 37–43.

Eddington, A. S. *The Nature of the Physical World*. Cambridge: The University Press, 1929.

Esslemont, J. E. *Bahá'u'lláh and the New Era*. London: Bahá'í Publishing Trust, 1974.

Fromm, Erich and Ramon Xirau. *The Nature of Man*. New York: Macmillan, 1968.

Jeans, Sir James. *The Mysterious Universe*. Cambridge: Cambridge University Press, 1931.

de Mille, Agnes. *Martha: The Life and Works of Martha Graham*. New York: Random House, 1991.

Peck, M. Scott. *The Road Less Traveled: A New Psychology of Love, Traditional Values and Spiritual Growth*. New York: Simon & Schuster, 1978.

Petersen, Ronald C. *Mayo Clinic on Alzheimer's Disease*. New York: Kensington Publishing Corporation, 2002.

Scheffler, Harlan Carl. *The Quest: Helping Our Children Find Meaning and Purpose*. Oxford: George Ronald, 2006.

Teilhard de Chardin, Pierre. *The Phenomenon of Man*. New York: Harper Perennial, 1976.

Zander, Rosamund Stone and Benjamin Zander. *The Art of Possibility: Transforming Professional and Personal Life*. New York: Penguin Books, 2006.

References and Notes

1. Petersen, *Mayo Clinic*, p. 175.
2. Esslemont, *Bahá'u'lláh and the New Era*, p. 209.
3. 'Abdu'l-Bahá, *Selections*, p. 48.
4. Teilhard de Chardin, *Phenomenon of Man*, book 4, ch. 2, p. 265.
5. Esslemont, *Bahá'u'lláh and the New Era*, p. 209.
6. Jewish-born humanistic philosopher, social psychologist, 1900–80.
7. Fromm and Xirau, *Nature of Man*, p. 306.
8. Eldest son of Bahá'u'lláh, founder of the Bahá'í Faith, 1844–1921.
9. See 'Abdu'l-Bahá, *Some Answered Questions*, pp. 208–9, 242–3; and 'Abdu'l-Bahá, *Tablet to August Forel*.
10. Petersen, *Mayo Clinic*, p. 14.
11. 'Abdu'l-Bahá, *Some Answered Questions*, pp. 24–6.
12. ibid. p. 239.
13. American dancer and choreographer, 1894–1991.
14. Martha Graham, quoted in Zander and Zander, *Art of Possibility*, p. 116; and de Mille, *Martha*.
15. This challenge is addressed in my book *The Quest: Helping Our Children Find Meaning and Purpose*.

www.ingramcontent.com/pod-product-compliance
Lightning Source LLC
Chambersburg PA
CBHW032014190326
41520CB00007B/464